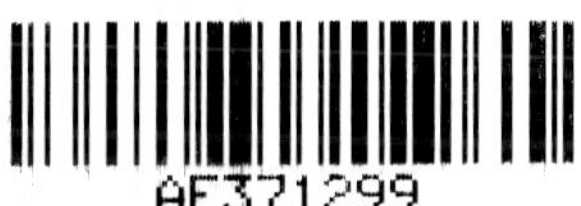

Made in the USA
Monee, IL
08 January 2025

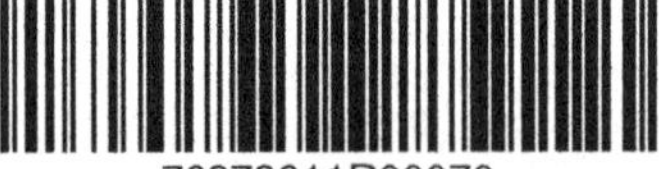